Making Your Donations Count

by

Susan Devine Napoli

To: The givers and the helpers.

Contents

***

Introduction

This is the third installment of a series on eating healthy, one I did not expect to write. I read the other two books today to get a perspective on what you might see as you read one to the other. There is a decline in them that is intentional and I want you to know that I am okay. Let me explain. Stress was building throughout the time period between August 2015 until now July 2017 in my life for reasons I did not know and came to find out. It got so intense that I finally threw my hands up in the air and said, "God, I can't do this. You can have my business. I can't make it work."

That is all God wanted to hear. I had been following signs and urges and seeking something that ended up to be him. After that, he asked me to do some weird things I did not get. Willing to do them to get out of the mess I was in, proved to have blessings in them I did not expect. It was hard, amazingly hard and exceedingly loving.

It was time to do something with my business for others, write another book. It's what I do. It is what my business is about. I thought I was doing that already. He wanted to take it to a new level. I had no idea it would come together as it did. As I read the previous two books, I had no idea God was in the midst of those too. No wonder my doctor was surprised at the numbers. No wonder there is this tremendous creative flow going on. God had something to say through what I already loved to do.

In this book, he asked me to do things that wore myself down to be completely nutritionally deficient that I did realize what was happening and complained bitterly about it in my now comfortable relationship with God. Why God why? Now I know. I was to write the book in a place of weakness, broken feeling, and completely out of resources. It got to the point I was scared to drive, the nutritional deficiency had taken my judgement and made me feel irritable. I did not go out today with one day left.

He asked me to do that, to teach you something. Something I had the talent to write about what I was learning and hearing from God, to pass on to you. It is going to be a treat and a hard read. It is also a call to action in your new leveled up information. A call to take care of people better.

I am one small voice in a big world. Blessed be.

My Story

It was not in my plan to have to ask for help. What I found was that I had to, by design. I had never done so before. I relied on family and credit cards for that little bit it took to get by at the end of the month. I knew I was living on the edge. I felt like I could lose it all just like that. I actually did. As I mentioned before, it was by design, God's design.

I had been working toward a life I would love better than the one I had. I had read and heard so much about these individuals who did. I took a chance and went for it, a little at a time. The closer I got to it the harder it got. A successful person as a full time instructor in the community college, I knew what it took to get to something like this. The big surprise was this time I was being actively blocked from it. So here I was, asking for help.

Basically, I don't qualify for programs. I am in between. I also have work to do, my writing. It does pay a little bit once a month. Every dollar counts. I feel directed to by God to keep going and not get a part time job. Part of what I do is to give insight on the things I come up against and how it worked out. It is a collection of books on a wide variety of topics. One of those topics is how to make ends meet. To not only survive but thrive. I have gotten some incredible results that I am proud of. But better than that is the insight I got in the process.

I used to donate from my excess regularly. Mostly stuff the kids had outgrown, things from my own closet I did not want anymore. Food from my pantry I did not eat. Books to the book resale shop. I did so knowing that it could help someone, and maybe even me, one day. I had no idea that I actually would be <u>using</u> this treasure that I had stored in heaven.

However, I had no idea what it was like to be a recipient. I just kept giving of the excess I had. There was quite a lot of it. It took actual years to whittle it down to a manageable amount. Then the bottom fell out and I learned what I really needed to live...and it surprised me how little. It was tremendously freeing and easy to manage. Spring cleaning did not need to happen. Chores that took most the weekend, didn't either. Anymore. So here is what I found out when I accepted my first bag of groceries. I am a voice from the other side to guide to give you some ideas for the giving you want to do.

I am here to say that all giving of things one does not need, is good. I appreciate all of what I have been able to buy at very low prices and for free, just because someone gave. As with most things I write about, I put my own spin on it. Thank you for taking a look at this book. You are in for a treat.

This is not an experiment like some writers do. It is the real deal. I am a retired educator, turned writer. It is my gift to the world. I thought as I got my first bag of food, there must be something in it to share. There was. Right away ideas started coming and I wrote them down.

***

Who These People Are

There is quite a bit of misinformation out there about people in a jam like me. I was assigned to go on a United Way tour for work a few years ago and went to five places in a shuttle van with others. I was amazed how they could do so much with so little. I went to a food bank, a clinic in a school, a home for adults with special needs, a senior citizen center, and a thrift store. I found there was a network of these places all attached by computer. Nobody gets to "soak the system" anymore. The agencies talk to each other. Most of the people they serve are in temporary stuck spots they are working to get out of. They are not homeless and many are working minimum wage jobs. Or in between jobs. Some are elderly. Some are sick. Some are special needs who cannot fully take care of themselves. Some are people in a one-time jam like me. It is that little bit to get them through. All of these places run on prayer.

This book has five sections:

Food

Electronics

Clothing and Appearance

Shelter

Friendship

These are the essentials to survival. I include electronics not as a joke but a necessity. It is a paperless world out there. Having one's own computer or device to use on a free Wi-Fi is signal is essential to having the information they need. It gives them the independence they need, once they learn how. There are free classes available for those that need to learn. Good classes with patient people. The others are familiar with technology from school and don't have their own device.

Friendship is the other surprise one. It is a necessity for survival in ways most do not expect. It can mean the difference between doing okay and doing well. Friendships are necessary to one's well-being.

I am not on this leg of my journey for nothing.

I am going to make every moment count.

You can move from becoming a good and regular giver to a great one, with just a few small changes. It could mean the world to someone you may never meet and an opportunity at a new life by getting a few precious things they long for.

***

Food

So what do you do with the empty bag to fill for the local charities? They are basically looking for shelf stable foods that are dried or canned. It is pretty simple, or seems so.

Have you given thought to how what you give will be prepared? Have you given thought to the individual dietary needs of the people receiving it?

Look at your own budget and determine where the waste is. Some families waste more food than they eat. Honest. My household was one of them. I went grocery shopping weekly with the best of intentions. I got tired mid-week and then went out to eat the remainder of the week. The food in the refrigerator spoiled. I would throw it out and start again the next week. As I sat in my new dilemma, I realized something. I could still be eating what I had wasted from those days, now. I would <u>never</u> have had to go food shopping at <u>all</u> in the two years that I have lived currently if I had the food i threw out. This is not to scare you but to cause you to think about what you have and can give. Food waste is a terrible thing that others can eat from. All it takes is a bit of planning, one I did not have time for then. When I did have time, I was working on it slowly.

I have now written two such plans in books I have written:

<u>Healthy Cooking, Healthy Living on $176 a Month: my story</u>

And

<u>Power Foods for Stressful Times: the companion book</u>

Both books go into detail on how it is possible to eat heathy on a very small budget. Let me continue that discussion I have in there with some ideas for giving. Some are from the books and some are new to this one.

An old idea in American Kitchens is to have it well-stocked. I looked through many old cookbooks. It seems to come from a time when there weren't grocery stores and one had to put food away for the winter. It was also influenced by the great depression. To stock up. Those who have lived through it find it hard, even today, to not have it fully stocked. It is a sign of plenty and having made it, to have such a kitchen. It is not a problem if one eventually eats it all to the bare cupboards. My hunch is that it is probably not, as mine was.

I began to work on this problem on vacations, collecting recipes and developing lists of food we loved to eat. Then I would buy only the items on that list. It was the impulse buying that got to me. I would buy four when I needed only two. The extra two could have gone in the donation bag. I am not talking about a lot here, just the little bit that is too much. Many families would not even feel such a donation to give to their favorite distribution site.

There is a discomfort to many Americans to have empty cupboards. It is a social stigma that either one is in a lot of trouble or a joke of a single man or college student. It really could be a lifestyle to not waste, anymore.

When one wants to give it is important to consider the health of the individual who would receive such a gift of food. The distribution sites can only give what they get. They cannot give the gift of healthy eating if they don't receive it. Bit by bit Americans are figuring out how to eat healthy and not buying the foods that lead to health problems. Food has a big role to play in the health of individuals. The cheaper foods are going into the donation bag. It seems like a good idea...I did it too. It isn't.

Many individuals who receive this food are serving. That is good. What they want is clear skin, hair, and nails like those who eat better have. They want the opportunity to lose a few pounds. They want to be clear headed. What they have is high blood pressure, prediabetes, heart disease, and a whole host of health problems that stem from the Standard American Diet. Those who are especially at risk are those who have to eat from the Standard American Diet long term like many of these people do. They want to eat the healthy foods and feel good. They want a chance to thrive. Having looked around at many of the diseases, the dietary needs are similar: whole foods as close to nature as possible, no processed foods. Consider the following in your donation bag:

Small bottles of olive oil

Vegetables packed in low salt

Fruits packed in low sugar or fruit juice

Dried fruits

Whole grain products, like popcorn and dried grains

Nuts

Soy milk, nut milks

Canned beans, dried beans

Canned meats and fish

Dried seasonings: to make hummus with, enhance the flavor of the foods

Ready-made sauces and broths to add meat and vegetables

Brown rice noodles and crackers

Isn't that expensive? No. I bought the cheapest of these type of items in the store brands, WIC foods (a foods program for women, infants, and children selected nutritious foods marked and sold at every grocery store), and the dollar store. I turned my health around for the first time in a decade eating these "cheap" but nutritious foods. If you really look, you can get one of each other these items for a dollar, the total cost would be $15 of the previous list for someone in need, 15 items of good health.

Why would you want to do that? Because a healthier person is a more productive one. One that can get out of the mess they are in because they don't <u>have</u> to live and work through high blood pressure or a diabetic fog. Food in the Standard American Diet sends them to bed. A napping person is not a productive one. It helps to break the cycle to donate with their dilemma in mind.

Standard American Diet

I have a list and a discussion of what processed foods are and what they did to my heath on page 77 in the healthy cooking, healthy living book. If you have never "wrestled with a candy bar", I invite you to read about it on page 10 of the Power Foods Book. Why am I not listing those here? Because I want you to read the books and then put them in the donation bag or make them available in the library at the donation site, free of charge to those who need it. The need is greater for those who live on limited incomes to get this kind of information. Nothing beats a free book or two. This book is for you to become savvy in your giving. It is not about selling books either but meeting needs, one at a time.

Let me give you one tempting piece bit of knowledge. I have been praying and following God's direction closely as I can, during the time from November until July. In November I moved to my current apartment in a panic. By the end of November, I had gotten the directions in my prayer time for the power food changes. It took one month to feel remarkably better and then two more to feel amazing. I ate nothing but the fresh foods that I listed in the book. When February came I was given the directions to add in eating out. Then March I ate out some more adding fast food. Then April was even more eating out. Then May, I found myself depleted and I was given very specific directions to add orange vegetables: butternut squash and carrots. Right away I perked up and stopped being dizzy in two days' time and ate other heathy foods. In June, I felt so good that I ate birthday cake. Then chips and dips days later. I felt good. I ate one of everything I hadn't had in months and years. In July, I ate the food that took me to the doctor in 2009, I was completely miserable. Mid-month, I started to run out of food. Trusting God, I knew that he would supply my need. The last week of the month I was told to go ask for help. I never did before. What I did get was a bag of groceries of food I knew I should not eat. I am bloated and take naps after I eat. It is four days until pay day where I wil get back to the power foods for keeps. I am counting the days. I am miserable once again. I have been wondering about all the changes. This is what happens to people on the Standard American Diet and eating good foods when it is not consistent. It is a roller coaster ride. I visited with my son and he is concerned that my memory is failing. Nope, it is what happens when people do not get to stay on the healthy diet of whole good foods. It is something people can commit to for those who need it the most. If they get that opportunity, the nutrients would work their power almost right away. As someone who eats healthy like me, it would take longer for your body to become depleted since the nutrients are stored.

Of course I am assuming you eat healthy, lots of people eat the Standard American Diet out of habit and not wanting to bother with it. Lots of people think they have a problem with losing weight on this diet. Try as I might, small meals on this diet will not allow you to lose weight unless you count and measure. Your body thinks you are starving and you might gain weight. I gained 15 pounds in three months. There is something to this power food diet and other like it that center on vegetables, lean meats/beans/nuts, and seasonings including lemon, tomato based sauces, balsamic vinegar, ponsu sauce, and dried herbs. It has infrequent dairy and breads/whole grains. These are a treat. Desserts are berries and tiny amounts of sweet like frozen yogurt and chocolate covered fruit. I lost about 30 pounds eating this way without measuring any food. I felt good. I felt strong. I felt clear headed. My skin stopped breaking out.

There are many who are trying to put a stop to the Standard American Diet. Consider doing your part in the food drives you donate to. Although the people will be forced to eat this way, it won't be long to see they do not have to be rich to be healthier, just richer in information they don't have.

Prayer

As someone who donates, I want you to consider to pray for those you donate to. It is a tough thing to get a bag of food items and try to figure out how to prepare it. That is why I want you to put the books in the bag to have simple recipes to spur their ideas. It is not an easy thing to figure out what to do and takes much longer than going to the store and getting what you want to eat. Have you ever have a can of baked beans and a can of corn for a meal? I have. It was my best option. Consider donating items that complete each other like not butter and crackers or lean meat and vegetables. Consider to never ever donate again from what you will not eat yourself. It seems like a good idea, it isn't. These people are not less than, they are real human beings like you and me who deserve a real chance, not get stuck in a cycle they cannot get out of.

One other idea is this: consider having the shopping services at grocery store shop your donation of these foods. That way it can save you time and it takes minutes to pick it up or have it delivered to the donation site. A click of the mouse and you have done a great deed for the month. If enough people request these foods to donate, the demand will go up, making them easier to find and the stores will stock them. They are a business and business goes with what sells. It is a lot like voting in that manner. You have more power than you think to change a life for the better.

Growth

Eating well helps children too, it develops their brain for school. They do get support from WIC, but it is only a supplemental plan. It doesn't feed them all day, every day. They have to get food stamps for that. Then the choices are theirs on what to feed their children. The WIC office is great about the support they offer. They weigh the child and give him or her a checkup by a nurse practitioner. The health of the mom is looked at too. It is a combination of services that help the mothers, infants, and children. Few programs go beyond age two. I had one Dad come by my office at the college where I worked, and ask me. They needed help and their child was two. The local Women's Crisis center helped them for one more year. They had an education program where they could earn diapers and formula and free babysitting while the parent learned. The amount of videos and classes they attended became "baby bucks" to cash in for what the parents needed for their baby.

It takes a team to grow a healthy baby into a child ready for school and the world. Parents are not always knowledgeable but it would not be a first assumption. It is safer to assume they do, and don't have the resources. Anyone's life can fall apart, anyone's. A lack of resources does not mean they don't know what to do, it means they can't.

Growth for the adults is harder to come by. There are a few programs for adults I know about, mostly at the community college. What they offer can vary in cost. I live between two community colleges. Both offer GED classes, one at nearly $300 a course, the other is free for the same thing. The free courses are in an area of greater need. They only charge for the test which is less than $100. At the other college they pay for the four classes and then the test for the same thing. There are testing services and placement into basic adult education starting at about the fourth grade level and continues through the credit program to earn training certificates and associate degrees. Of course the price goes up as the achieve more. The FASFA program is grant money, free money to go to school. As is the Pell Grant. Grants they don't have to pay back and some money is set aside for them to earn as a student worker on campus.

The community college also had continuing education classes for people who want to learn for fun. Sometimes these classes are mixed in with the regular college students. Sometimes they meet just once. Most people think that the community college is just like high school, 13th and 14th grades. Actually, they stand in the gap between having a hard time in school to earning a degree that could feed them and theirs for a lifetime. The age varies from age 16 to senior citizens. Many people in mid-life think they will be the oldest one in the classes and on campus but they have lots of company. he community college is a unique system in which they get real college, connections, and experiences for a career.

Libraries offer adult classes depending on who they can get to come teach. They have staff on duty to teach computer skills at no cost. There is also a media room and a creative space that has machinery like the 3D printer and laser cutter. They are open to speakers to share what they like to do. It is easy to get on the schedule. The content and the level varies a lot. The classes tend to be recreational in nature. It is for fun.

Churches stand in a different gap. They offer support for where these other programs do not.

They offer spiritual guidance and emotional support. They teach in sermons and offer companionship with no other goal. There are fun activities to do at little or no cost in some churches.

All of these program are not created equal, it depends on the dedicated folks who give their time and talent to it. Eating healthy foods allows people to participate in the programs with a clear head and happier outlook. I have seen people attend college classes at night after working all day, just to have chips and soda for "dinner". For some it is a time factor. For others, it is seen as a temporary condition until they graduate.

Hunger can make people demanding and crabby and do things they would not. Few people want to admit they are hungry or had to eat something that makes them lethargic and foggy headed, to try and make their life better.

Some refuse because of how they are treated, like with pity or seen as messed up. They would rather go hungry than be treated like that. Children are sensitive to it too. I had the opportunity to eat a free hot lunch while in high school. I refused, telling my mom I would rather eat anything than to stand in the special line. I was told I would have to eat peanut butter sandwich and an orange every day. And that was just what I did. Sometimes she got sliced meat. Sometimes the bread was older than the week before depending on what she could find. Sometimes I did get money for hamburger day, homemade back then, that had its own line and all the cool kids ate that every day. It was the happy meal size burger with a small French fries and an 8oz chocolate shake, not fast food. Food matters to kids. It matters to parents and adults of all ages. Everyone wants to eat the cool food. Right now it is fresh fruits and vegetables and lean meats. What could be better than that? They are waiting. They know that a boundary is there...help them cross, won't you?

***

Something for the Grocery Stores to Consider

Finding nutritious foods in a grocery store for a dollar or less is a hard thing, right now. My idea for you is to dedicate some shelf space to each section of your store for nutritious food items for just these type of items. Place them in the designated space and restock often. Just because a person has only $5 to spend does not mean they need a puzzle to go with it. If it is 10 for a dollar, it is easy to think they have to buy ten when they do not. The wording "$1, limit 10" is clearer. Everyone likes to run in and get what they want and leave to be on to other things in their lives, everyone. Including those living dollar to dollar.

What you would be doing is taking the guess work out of it too, providing small portion sizes for the college student, the retiree, the person in a bind, and the tight wad too. Make it inviting. Make it all out war with your competitors by having the best stocked dollar sections. The need is greater than you think. People should have more choice than what the dollar stores can offer.

Have friendly people near these sections to assist, really friendly. The dollar stores has you beat hands down on this. They honestly do. Go stealth at you local dollar store and see. Nobody gets put down there, ever for what they buy or how they pay. No one gets asked about why they purchased what they did. No one ever has a clerk down their neck hurrying people who clearly need a moment to fumble with their payment. Kindness is better than speed in the long run. It will give you more customers of the right kind. The customers who are in a huff and a hurry will take their business elsewhere to grump and grumble at people who are in need there. Don't worry, they will be back when the bottom falls out for them and glad for your smile. It happened to me. I was one of the grumpy entitled ones. It should not be so hard to find and buy low cost, highly nutritious food. It shouldn't. Especially when it is there in the store already.

Electronics

Getting electronics is difficult for some. Easy to get and hard to keep. The companies are very large and have no problem with cutting service. They have many customers. This makes this in between population very vulnerable to having multiple phone numbers over a period of time. Email they cannot get at. Accounts they cannot access because it is hooked up to an old phone number. These devices are traceable with a GPS and Bluetooth by even the novice with a computer. It can present safety issues for some when the bottom falls out of their lives and harassment, intrusion, and demands come one after another. A donation of electronics allows people to start again by owning their own device for a reasonable price.

By the direction of God and the TV remote, I turned it on and found a repeat of a program I had seen months earlier. I knew that there were refurbished electronics for sale somewhere at a store. I did not know the name or the location. After looking over the area, I was not satisfied with what I could get locally. I came home and turned on the TV, there was the program I had seen before and the name of the store...Goodwill. I learned they take donations of electronics, give people a job refurbishing them and put them up for sale at reasonable prices. The next day I was directed to go and find the address of this shop. I found there were several. I planned my route. The inner directions were 'get $150 cash and go tomorrow'. It was a trusting experience I was not sure of. How would I know that was enough money? How would I know they had what I needed? I didn't. I didn't even have phone service to check or a GPS to help me find the store. I was going on blind faith.

I got lost twice. I got directions from two kind people and ended up thankful at the store. I knew I needed a laptop to continue my writing that people wanted me to stop. I needed a laptop to work offline. I had mistakenly bought an online only computer. I did not want to work in the cloud and have the opportunity for my writing to be compromised. I had foolishly bought a computer without asking God. Now he was giving me one. When I got to the Goodwill electronics store, I was directed to two laptops. One that looked like the one I had, so I chose the other one for $122. I was so thankful. The beautiful woman that sold it to me and answered my questions set me at ease. She showed great care with everything. Though she didn't say, I think she refurbished it herself. She had a soft pride in her work. I paid her and ate lunch on the way home with the remainder of the money. God is good. I felt so loved.

I checked out my computer and I realized it was more of a blessing than I thought. It did not need to be registered like a new computer does. That offered me a level of safety over my work I did not expect. I was extremely grateful. I did a test on a document and it saved. The next day I found it to be compatible with the library computer for uploading my work. It took a little while to adjust to an older model of a really good computer. It even charges faster than the new one. I began calling it God's computer. He made it possible to work anywhere. My work is a stealth kind of operation that I did not intend it to be. People think that I am online when I am writing.

A donation of old electronics to Goodwill are handled with great care. They take all kind of electronics to refurbish. Desk computers. Electric Guitars. Everything. These would be perfect for students on a budget who can get the software they need for free at school sometimes. Laptops are particularly in demand. Through my experience I would have no problem with donating old electronics at all. After I had seen the first show on the TV, I also saw the story of Goodwill in Houston, where I live. It started as a place to train people with special needs. Today it is a place that will give a job to anyone who is in any kind of need. There was a woman on there who lost her husband and had no means to take care of herself. She now works at Goodwill in the office. Goodwill need workers of all abilities and talents. I realized I would have qualified too based on my circumstances. Someone with a master's degree like me would get to work in the corporate offices or something suitable for my abilities. I did not apply, though sure that I would get a job. I had work to do for God with my computer. I would not hesitate one moment to donate anything to Goodwill. They saved me more than they will know.

Service for electronics is limited to free Wi-Fi in restaurants and many other public places that one can have for the price of a cup of coffee, cheaper than one's own service. It is a great service but it is shared, much like the party lines of phones of not that long ago in America. My bank account has been breached twice. I closed the cards. I did not type the number on Wi-Fi, it was already in there. The breech involved taking control of my account even though I only used the computer at the bank for my banking. There was no fraud. It pays to be vigilant with the help of the Holy Spirit.

The connected society is a comfort for some and a nightmare for others. This maybe hard understand for some but if you do the work of God, you are going to come up against opposition. Some of it will be electronic. They will look you up and take you down from the comfort of their own home. God knows this, he made a way for me to be connected without service. Only the bold will attempt something in person. Mostly they don't need to as the electronic will take care of it. Unregistered electronics are not traceable if they never go online and the Bluetooth and GPS is off.

This information needs to go to those in domestic violence and other scary situations to help people escape. They have to be untraceable. They cannot post on social media, which gives away their location. If they shut off the location, photos they post could give clues to where they are and what they are doing. It is also way too easy to trust the wrong person during a time like this and mistakenly give away clues. It is important for these people to follow the directions of the Holy Spirit during this time. Your donation of electronics could save a life, quite literally.

God knows exactly how the electronics work. He can make devices "fail" when they are fine. He can make them "work" when they are not connected correctly. The message will get to where it need to go at the time it is to go there. He will make delays happen and instantaneous go faster. He can create interference. I have never once missed an important message. I get tips to go check from him. It is surprising how few of them are really important in the tidal wave of information I used to look at. He likes that much better.

When I mean interference, I am referring to a specific incident one morning at a meeting, the first meeting of the year back to work in the auditorium. I struck up a conversation with the man next to me I had met years earlier and never seen since, seven years later. The program began right away and then surprisingly, there was some kind of interference with the audio visual equipment. We just kept talking. I felt a spark of something between us. It was what is called a glimpse. I felt and heard something like a call from the future and possibilities opened for me. He let me know later in the program when I laughed way too loud and softened it, he put his arm against mine. That cemented the glimpse and the calling in my mind. Overwhelmed, I did not say anything else. When the meeting was over, I went to my office and smiled for the first time in years. I had gone in to work to quit my job that morning. I decided to stay and see what this was all about. That is what I mean when I say that God uses seemingly inconvenient things to happen. Had the equipment not "failed" we would never have had the conversation that lead to the glimpse. Even at work. At the end of the program, I was sitting close enough to the front to hear the audio guys. One remarked to the other, "I don't understand it. It worked just fine earlier this morning." I do, and did at the time. It was so church could happen for me at work. I was too stubborn to ever go to church on my own. God brought it to me that day.

So that is why donating electronics is so important to those in need. God can speak to them through having a device or two of their own. He can lead them that way in unconventional ways and love them in a modern manner that we are accustomed to today.

***

Clothing and Appearance

One of the first indication to others that something is not going right is the change in one's appearance. Hair and clothing are the first things people notice and will ask about. It is a sign to be doing well to have hair neatly cut and new clothes periodically. It doesn't have to be fancy, just tended to regularly as to not gain unwanted attention.

Hair styling is real important to people and is cultural in some cases. Missing hair care can be devastating to the one who knows they need it. It can be very dramatic for those who choose to color or perm or straightened and their hair goes back to being natural. It is hard to wait for it to grow out with nothing they can do about it.

In my case it was a simple cut and the big change was length. It grew until it caught under my arm pits. I realized I needed a haircut and thought of my favorite place to get it cut was not out of reach. They charge more for length. My simple cut was now $90 to work with. I was horrified. Someone asked me how long was it since I had a haircut? I got to thinking about getting it done as cheaply as possible. Then it dawned on me...beauty schools. Yes, they need practice and I had nothing but time. I looked them up and a cut was $15. I went to get it cut and got a nervous new student. It took her nearly two hours to put in long layers, a 20 minute cut. Her instructor did most of it. I looked fantastic. I went by six months later and she cut it again all on her own in 20 minutes. Patience pays. They discount the supplies more than other places that sell them. Beauty schools are everywhere. At community colleges, at vocational schools, at high schools, in shopping plazas. It would be cool to throw a gift card or two from such a place in your donation bag. The one I go to sells them. Look around, it would mean the world to someone.

Another part of personal appearance is one's clothing. Thrift shops like Goodwill and so many others have a large selection usually organized by color and th type of clothing it is. Goodwill is very good at that. They offer discounts to several groups of people who all they have to do is show their ID. Every day there is a color of the day that is reduced. The little plastic tag on the clothing together with ID can make a heavy bag of clothes, I have gotten as much as twelve pieces for $50.

Finding something wearable is another matter. No one likes to have outdated clothing. It creates attention no one likes.

Here is what I look for at thrift shops. Name brands. These are the brands that are at the local mall. The brands that no one questions. I look for tags of the item donated without being worn. Everyone likes new. I found a t-shirt from the Reba Collection at Dillards, never worn. It was easily a $80 shirt new there, I got it for $5. There are other savvy shoppers like me. One has to go often and with something in mind they are looking for in the color they like, it goes quicker that way.

Another thing I do is alter the clothing. Some of it is tossed aside because it has an annoying feature to it that looks bad on everyone. Because I can sew, I can alter it to suit me in a way that is cheaper than fabric. Amazingly cheaper. Once I figured this out, I was not embarrassed to buy clothing there anymore. I could alter it until it became my own design. I wrote books on how to do this. They are titled: <u>Altered Couture: my adventure In sewing</u> and <u>Practical Altered Couture</u> (coming soon). It is written for intermediate and advanced sewers or to be taken to sewing lessons. It has photos of the garments and the story that goes with it. It saves a lot of money so I could buy new underwear and shoes and socks. Essentials I will not compromise on.

Shelter

I wanted to find cheap housing that I could still have my studio to work in too. Separate site. The plan was to get both for $800, one for work one for home. It turned out to be a horrible experience. Cheap housing actually costs more than conventional. They charge a lot for a little bit and use the leverage to insist on things one cannot afford as add ons. It did not help I drove up in a recent model Chevy Camaro, my actual car at the time. I could go on but let me suffice to say I am at neither place today and have a conventional apartment for a reasonable price with both my work and home under one roof.

I learned quite a lot of things in the process and wrote two books titled <u>Tiny Living: from 1,300 to 400 square feet</u> and <u>Environment Matters</u>.(coming soon). It has lots of tips on clutter clearing and downsizing. Good for anyone who wants to make a change, even if it is not that dramatic. I found the amount of stuff that I had cost money to keep, money I didn't have anymore. It had other costs too like how it held me back in ways I did not know and reprioritized. As my life changed, the stuff went out. I have been purging much more than I say in the book because I continued to for another year until I found my purpose. I am in the middle of my last purge, getting rid of the nostalgic items that are not so much anymore. I have lived into the moment that I am building a setting that is for who I will become. That kind of insight comes from quiet and prayer, no one knows that otherwise. I love this leveled up space idea.

As I let go of things, I got better at sending them to thrift stores and found some will even pick up if you call them. These items are sold and used to run special programs like the popular prom dress donation in which girls can choose a dress and attend prom who would not ordinarily get to. They help the shelters that house those who run in the night from domestic violence. Once all of that became real to me, I had no problem donating my things at all.

As someone who gives and helps, clearing your home of things you don't remember what is in the boxes or the attic, can make a big difference to someone. It is an opportunity for those who must shop there, get the opportunity to choose items for themselves. Please do not hesitate to donate new items. It feels a little like a special occasion to find one or two to have something new and up to date.

***

Friendship

People can go through life with no one ever knowing their dream. They are afraid to let people know how "out there" it is. They go through the motions of life with it tugging at their heart, afraid that if the reveal it they will be rejected. That what they hold most dear will be torn to shreds. That if they reveal it, they will lose the very thing that they breathe for. The hope of it seems to be better than the fear of losing it. Most dreams develop in stages with starts and stops. It can be very hard to find someone who knows that.

Oprah Winfrey at the beginning of her talk show career, could not get a celebrity to interview on her show. She decided to go with what she had, regular people with their story. It was an instant success. In just a few shows she was wealthy beyond measure. It is not the money story so many think it is, she did something extraordinarily different. She listened. She listened in a world that does not. People listen to get a turn to talk, which is not listening. She listened and got all of the story, not just the part they wanted to reveal. It set people free who were watching and the people she was interviewing. It was a remarkable move, that I am sure was inspired by God. She is open about her faith. After that, everyone wanted to be one her show, including celebrities. They all wanted to be heard.

In my world no one listens. Even a little bit of telling one's story causes them to flee. Being sent to a therapist does not work either, their job is to heal the sick. The really sick, lost inside of themselves with chronic, and unalterable mental health issues. Many of their clients are people who are not suffering that way. They just need to be heard. To be able to tell the whole story and walk away from the pain. It is in telling that the pain stops. It is inherently bad to sit in an office and tell your story and then be cut off because time is up and to write a check. That is not listening, even though it appears to be. The manner they are trained to listen in is remarkable, but true caring is what adds to the listening experience. That is what Oprah did. That is what you can do too, offer the opportunity to someone to hear their story. To give the donation of time.

Time is a commodity that people wrestle with. They want to save it. They want to manage it. They want to control it. While they are figuring that out, it ticks on. They lose what they want to save, manage, and control. A gift of time to listen is what many people need. It costs nothing.

Let me suffice to say this: no one has ever heard my story. Not the whole thing. Not with the grace and love I hope for it to be received in. That is not different or strange, it is life for many. People shut down when they feel they are being judged. People shut down when they find their story becomes gossip. People shut down when they are made to feel less than because of it. No one gets through this life unscathed. Telling one's story is how they endure it. They have at least one friend that can really listen, like Oprah does. It is frightening how many people do not have that one person. It is frightening to know that in spite of the constant communication most people have only 2-4 people on their phones that they care about. When I heard that, it was an element in my teaching that I changed. I saw the cell phone scrolling as an escape.

I changed my teaching method to be active learning with problems to solve and people to connect with. The lecture was very short, mere instructions for how to do the activity and a little background information they could not get anywhere else. I had several activities for the class period. I took my cue from them that they did not know, when someone took the cell phone out I changed activities. When I did that, they would voluntarily put it away. I measured my success by how many times I saw the phones come out each class period. I sought to have zero but two was not bad either. I used the cell phones available as a resource. When we got stuck I would ask, "Does someone want to look it up?" It was surprising that someone usually did.

It made a people furious that I would expect then to engage in the activities, figure things out, do their work, support each other, and a whole host of things they did not expect. They wanted to eat lunch and be on their phones, in class. They wanted to hear what they already read and knew from the textbook. They wanted to be the one who knew the answers. I took away that opportunity. They did not know what was going on. It made them have to regroup and redefine for themselves what was happening. It was extremely threatening for them to have to connect in a world that does not connect, to go deeper in a world that wants the quick answer, and to find out that there was another way to learn. They did not want that. They wanted what was familiar and comfortable.

There were also those that loved it. It gave them the chance to be heard by the people at their table, to really learn the material and not memorize it. To belong. People started coming early and staying late, with me laughing a little and telling them they can stay if they want, I got to go home. It was transformative to a few, so much so their whole manner changed for the positive and even how they held their face and bodies. Needs were met by ordinary people to ordinary people.

Won't you consider the donation of time to listen? How would you do it? Start a group at church? Meet in the lounge at school? Put a little sign on your table at a coffee shop that says 'friend'?

Children got it covered. There are schools that have a friend bench. It is brightly painted and says "Friend" on it. If someone wants a friend, they go sit on the bench. The other children notice and go and invite the friend to play. I think it was invented by a child. It is the socially acceptable way to get a friend, by watching from a distance and waiting to be invited. The others see the need and the one who wants to meet it, voluntarily goes over to the child on the bench. It is ingenious how beautifully it works. There are friend benches in schools all over. It is much better than the teacher trying to match children. It doesn't work very well. I can attest to that. Where are the friend benches in the adult world? Nowhere.

People are sent to therapy when all they need is a friend. Not having a friend for a very long time can make normal people appear troubled, that are not. They are asked to pay for what is free in life. Adults do not make their unmet need known until it has piled up into something big and awful. They want to appear to have it together until it cracks and falls apart. All of it could have been made lighter or bearable by having one true friend.

Friend Center

My answer to this dilemma is to have a friend center. One in every community. It is not a place to get resources. It is the adult version of the friend bench. It has groupings of tables of all sizes for people to talk to each other over. It has pairs of chairs for the introverts and those who want to talk to one person. It has cold sodas and hot tea. It is a place to find and build friendships for those who have none. It is not a lonely hearts club or a place where the weird people go. It is for everyone who needs a friend to come and get one at no charge but the sodas and tea themselves, if that. It has real furniture, not plastic. It has hope plastered on the walls and care taken in everything that is done there. It is a place to tell the story of who they are. To be the friend that they have forgotten to be or figure out hoe it got lost. A place to laugh and cry and hope and dream. That is my dream of a friend center.

At age 58, it it too big of a venture for me to begin now. I have spent my whole adult life following and figuring this out that has been drawing me to it for years. I am looking for your help, to find a place in your community and use the ideas from my books as a starting point. It can be done. It can meet the unmet needs of those who, if they had a friend, would improve greatly. In small and simple ways they can help each other. My hope is in you. As for me, I will keep writing as long as I can to give fuel for friendships that come of it and hope to those to take on the venture of managing a friend center. It is going to be a lovely project that we will build together.

In Closing...

Once upon a time in my old life I taught a course called Family, School, and Community for teachers and child care providers and future administrators of child care programs. It was a course that scared me at first. I learned about the links in the community from my students who gave me glimpses of a few things that I wrote about in this book. I had no idea there was so much more until I lived it.

This book was written in love and not to offend. It is easy to make assumptions about people and their "situation". God in his infinite power and love gave me the inspiration to write it all down that sprung from a bag of food and so much more. I will always cherish that experience in the way it was given. It was such a blessing. It will make it easier in the future but not a lot, to ask again. Though I hope that I don't... as you might well understand. Know too that a little insight and education from someone who has "been there" can shed light on the giving and the helping God so loves. It can make you much more purposeful in what you choose to offer. God likes that even more to give with intention.

It is now only two days left on my count down until I get paid again.Thank you for your blessings and love. I am going to make it. Yes, I did write this book hungrier than usual. This time I think it was by design, God's. It is that way often the week before payday for me, yet this time it was extreme in lots of ways. I know too that my gift to you could be invaluable to others and go much further than I can reach alone.

One thing I did not mention was after I got home with the bag of groceries, something shifted in me later in the afternoon. It was the reassurance that my new life was ahead and I sensed a promise that went with it...the wordless kind. It said that I will forget all of this and it will feel like a bad dream, hard for me to remember. For a moment I got to feel the distancing of it and what it would be like for this troubling time to be in the long past. Neither the people that gave the food, nor the person who packed the bag, or the person who gave it to me could anticipate that. Me either. That is why we do things like this, for that intangible something that only God can give. That intangible something that changes as God changes things on our behalf.

My hope is big that you will take on at least one of these. The needs are great and the solution simple. Will it be healthy food? Old electronics? New clothing and haircuts? To have appropriate shelter and furnishings? To listen so that someone can tell their story? Or to open and manage a friend center in your community?

I will close with this quote I bought in 1980 at the university bookstore when I was away at school. I kept it until now. I never could figure out why I wanted it and kept it for so long. Today, it finally makes sense. I know for sure it belongs in this book. I can throw the yellowed mini poster away blinking away tears of joy. I finally found where it belongs.

"No one can do everything, but everyone can do something."

Do your something, whatever it is.

Thank you,

Susan

Prologue:

When pay day came I had to wait for the bank to open and get money to go food shopping. I had a list and things seemed to be normal. I had a tiny bit of protein shake for breakfast. By the time I finished shopping an inner alarm sounded. I needed to eat or I was going to faint. I ate a banana and walnuts. Then got an egg taco and Gatorade at the gas station. I ran some errands and things were going long. I had to excuse myself to go eat. The inner alarm went off again. I had a beef taco and some beans and guacamole. I skipped the rice and the tortillas. I had an apple. I thought I would bounce back quickly from this. Apparently not. It took a day longer and to follow my plan carefully.

I used to wonder about those who seemed to go to the emergency room so often in my neighborhood years ago. I did not understand it. With this new knowledge and experience I do more than ever. I could have had a ride to the emergency room today from this. Thankfully, I did not need it. I am so much more concerned about the plight of people eating whatever people give them and the effects of their bodies. This is really hard to come back from. Harder than I thought.

When I ate for $176 a month last year, people I knew felt sorry for me. I could not understand it. I felt better than I had in years. The food I ate were name brand and fresh. It was a consistent diet. I even had dessert from time to time, apple crisp. I had to watch it closely but I never felt like this. There is absolutely nothing wrong with eating on a very low budget if it is medium quality and fresh food. I cannot wait to go to back to being me and have my energy and drive to do what I love back again. I thank God for this experience. I heard in the quietness of the evening last night that I will never have to do this again. Just the same, there will be people who do. We have to serve them better, we just do. This is my plea for them as they sit in their silent stupor with almost no energy to dream a dream and their hope is out on the horizon.

Back Cover:

God loves it when you give to those in need. Have you given any thought to how it is being received? Is it _really_ making a difference? Maybe not so much. Here is a candid look through the eyes of one who has lived it for almost two years, a successful person by many standards, whose life fell apart. She found herself in a new world and gained insight on the plight of others. She has some ideas on how to upgrade and level up your giving in simple ways you never thought about. It takes a look at the following:

Food

Electronics

Clothing and Appearance

Shelter

Friendship

Her ideas are simple, yet challenge the common beliefs that any donation is a good one, those in need are soaking the system, and so many others that people think are true. It is a challenge to giving in a new way. You will never look at your donation bag the same again that begins with the question, "If this bag was mine, how would I use it?" You may be inspired to give with more intention, care, and love of your own resources in ways that may surprise you and the recipient you will never meet.